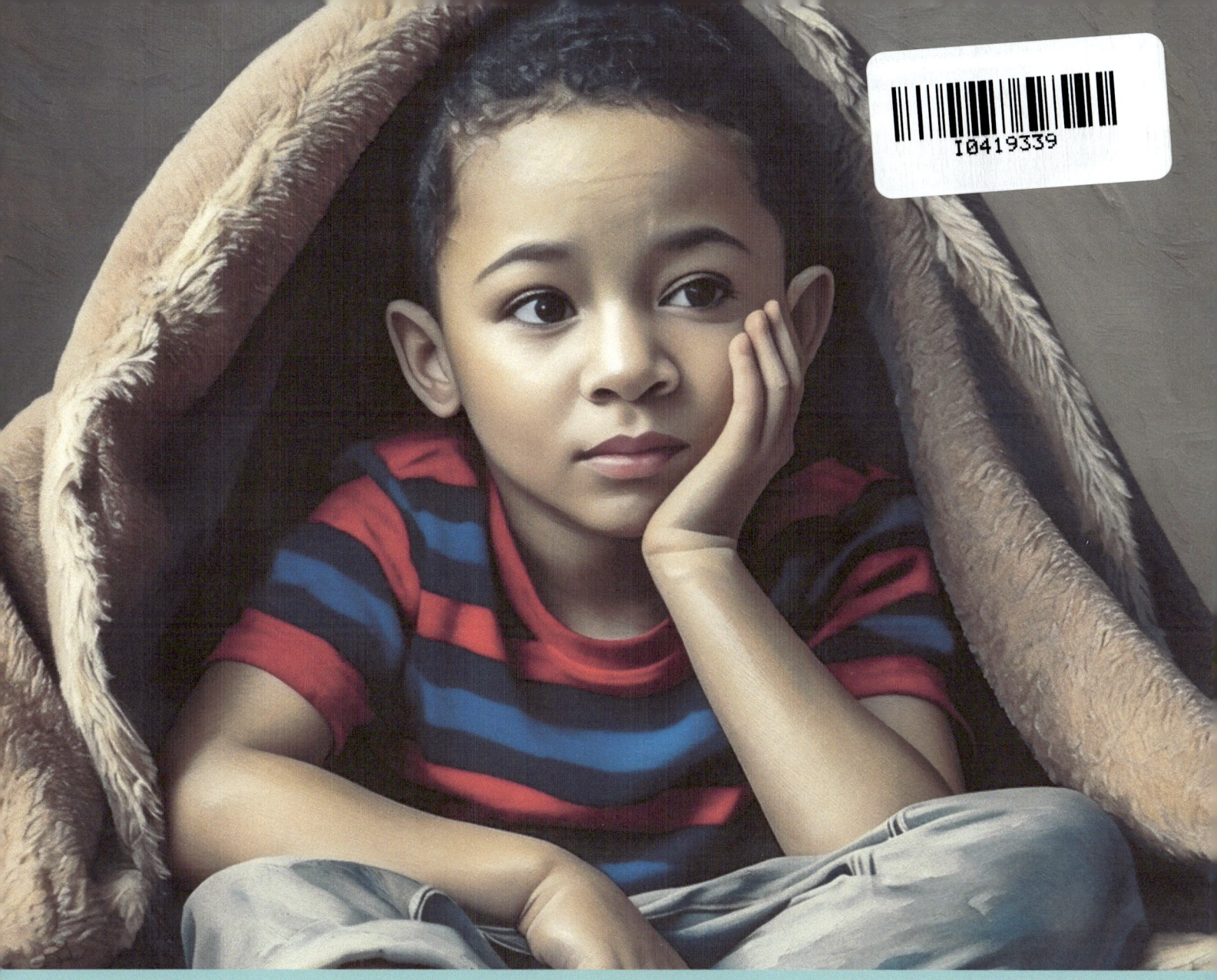

One day, Karsen started feeling really tired and thirsty.

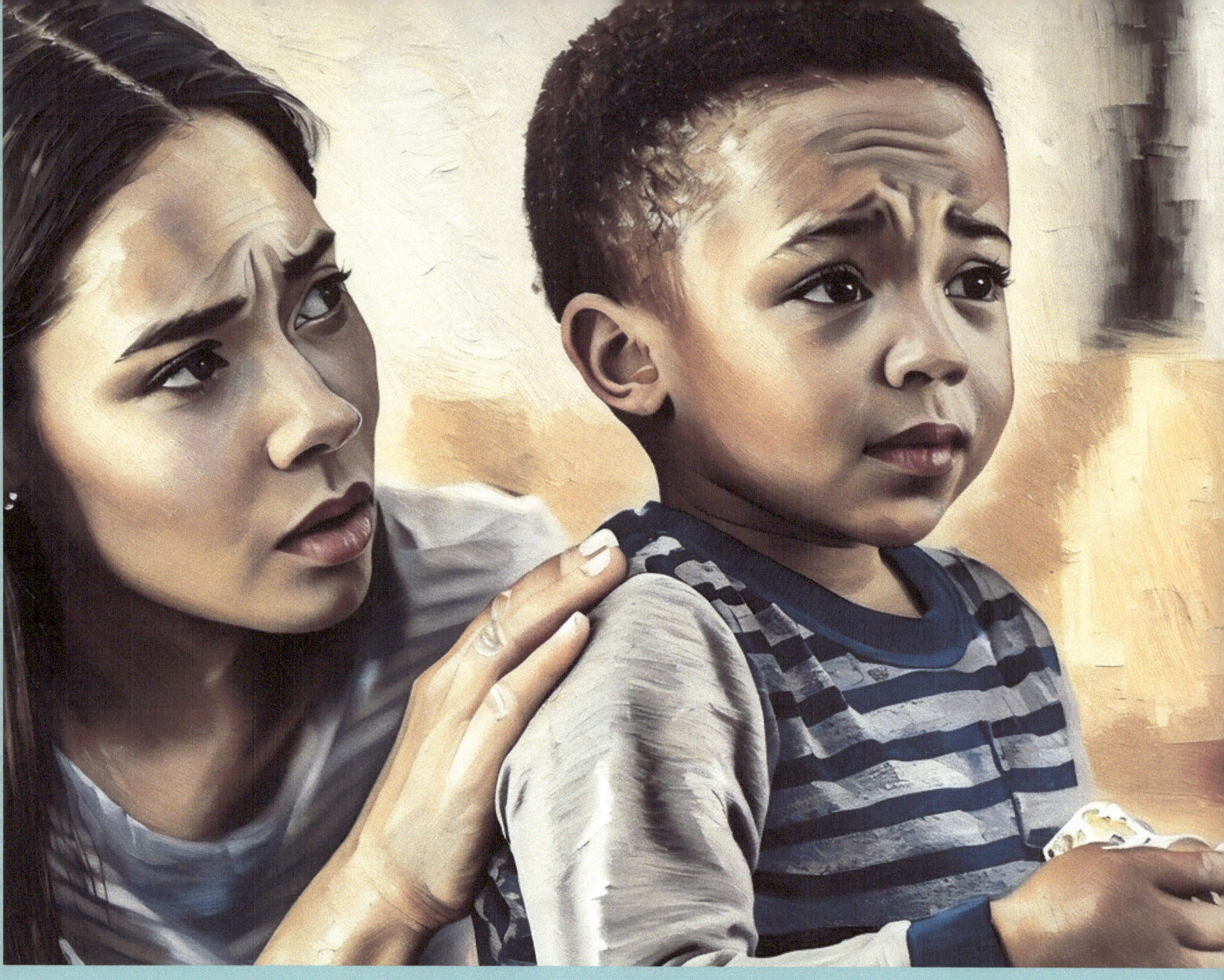

His mom noticed he seemed different than usual.

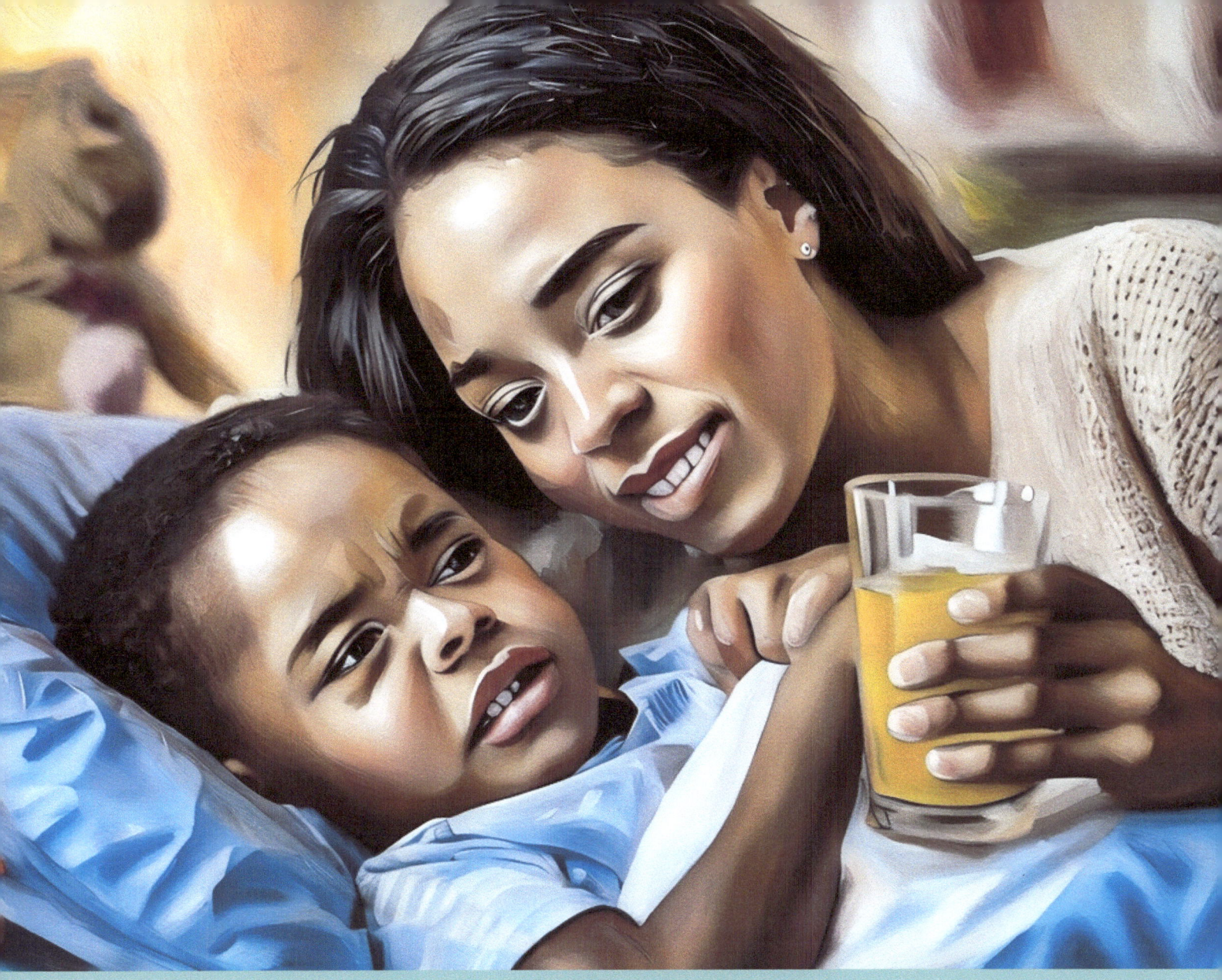

The next day, Karsen didn't feel like eating anything and he threw up the fluids he drank.

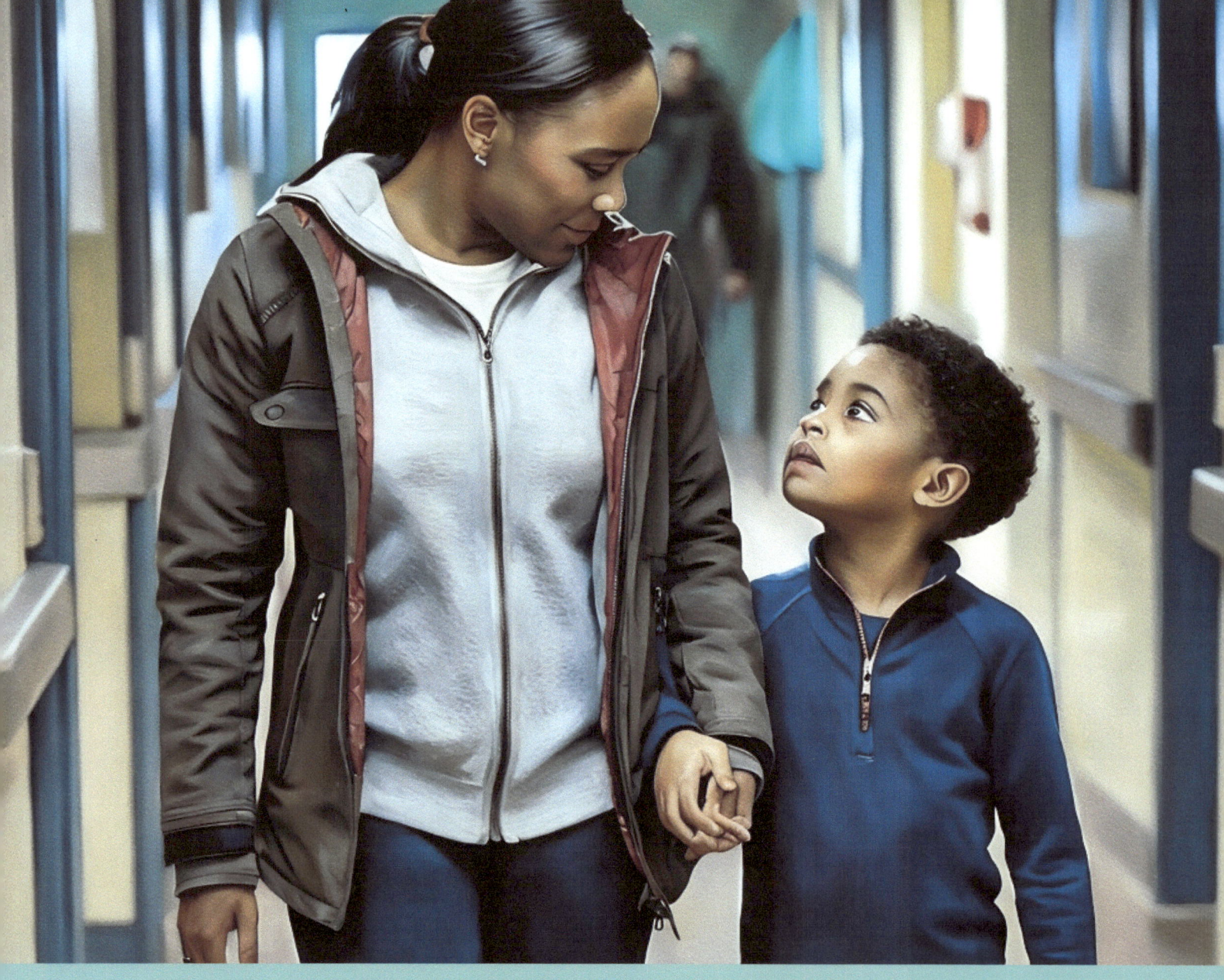

His mom took him to the hospital, saying, "No matter what happens, we will face it with courage."

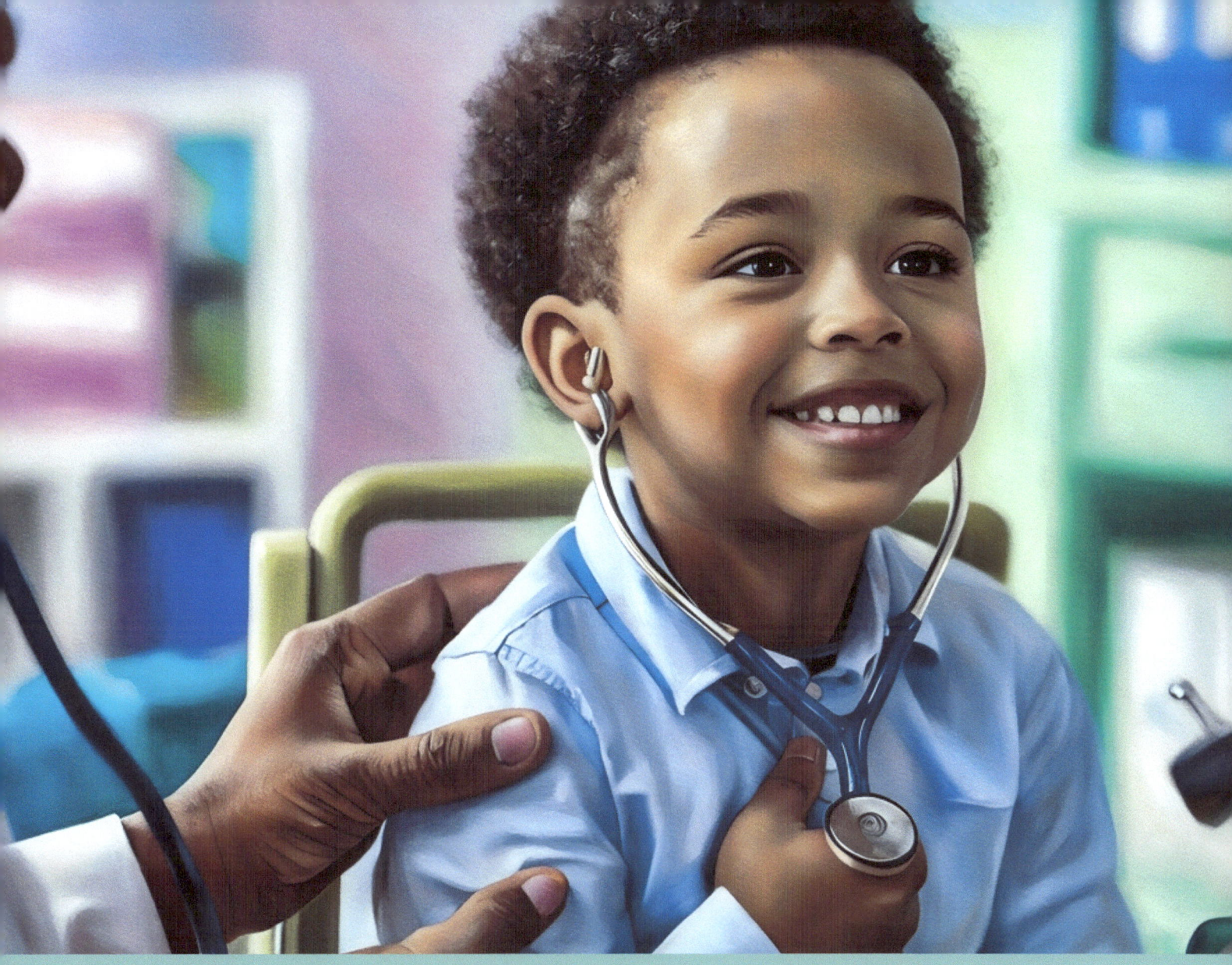

After receiving an examination at the hospital, the doctor said Karsen may be getting over a cold and could have a sore throat, which might explain why he didn't want to eat and threw up.

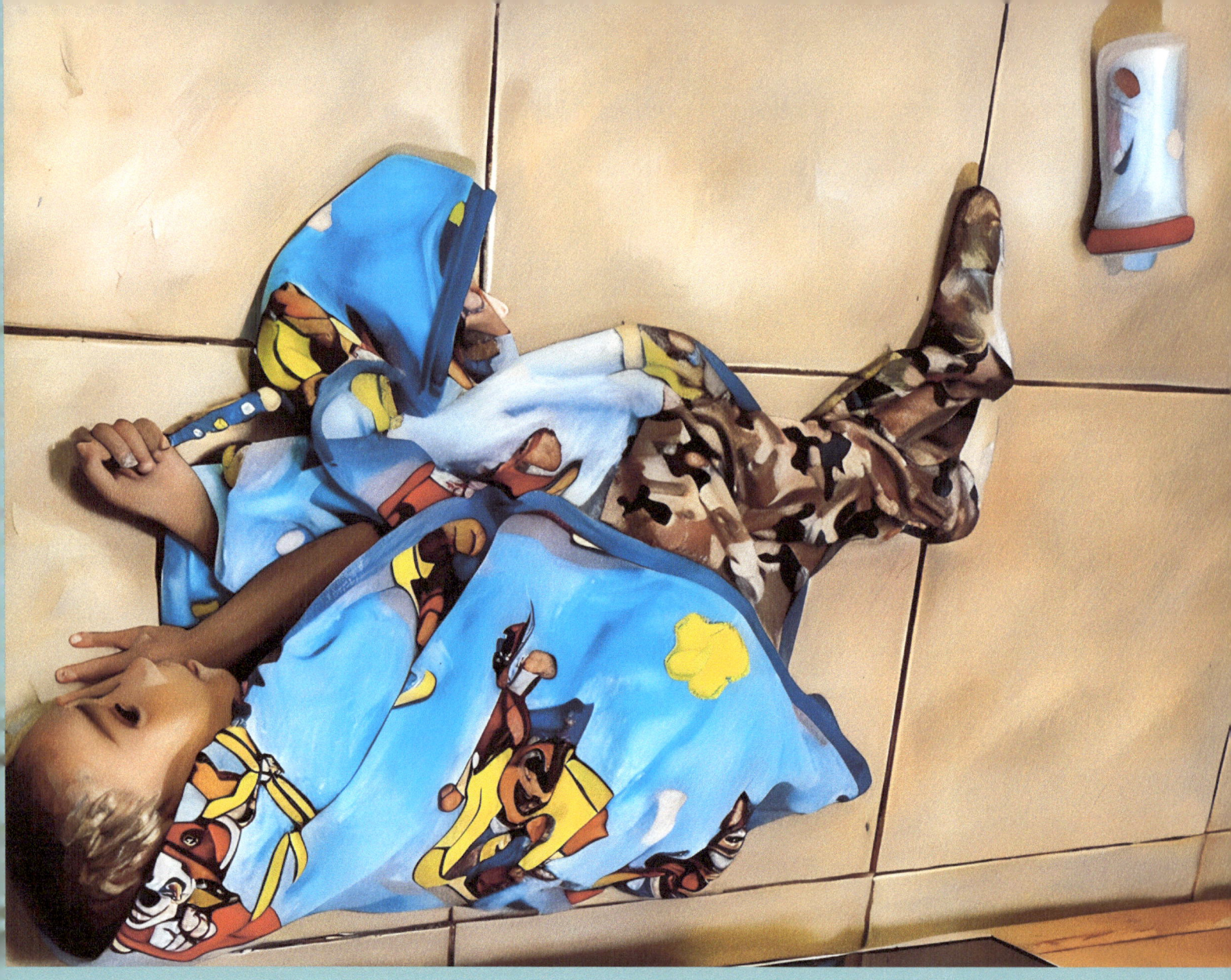

After leaving the hospital, Karsen's symptoms got worse.

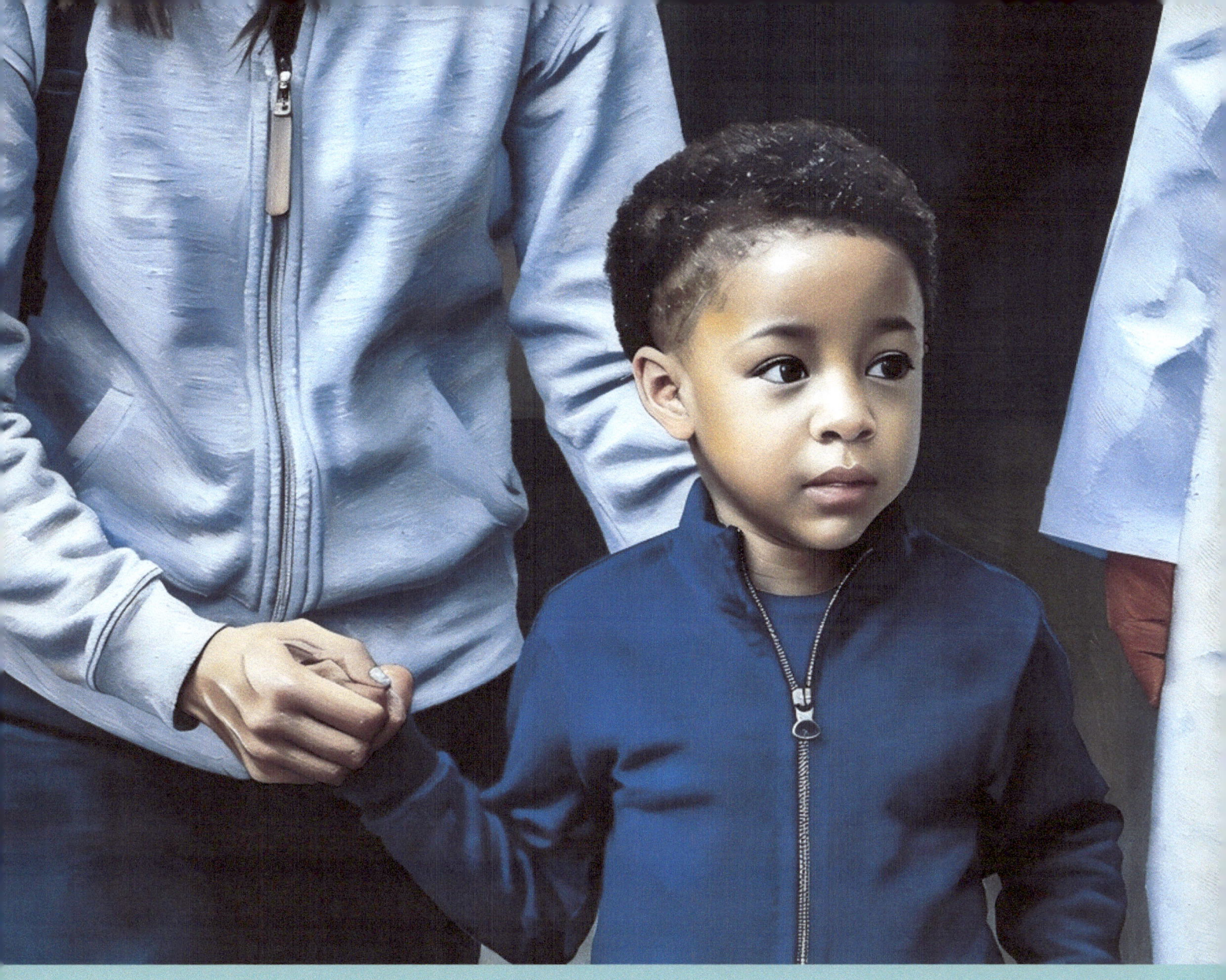

His mom took him back to the hospital.

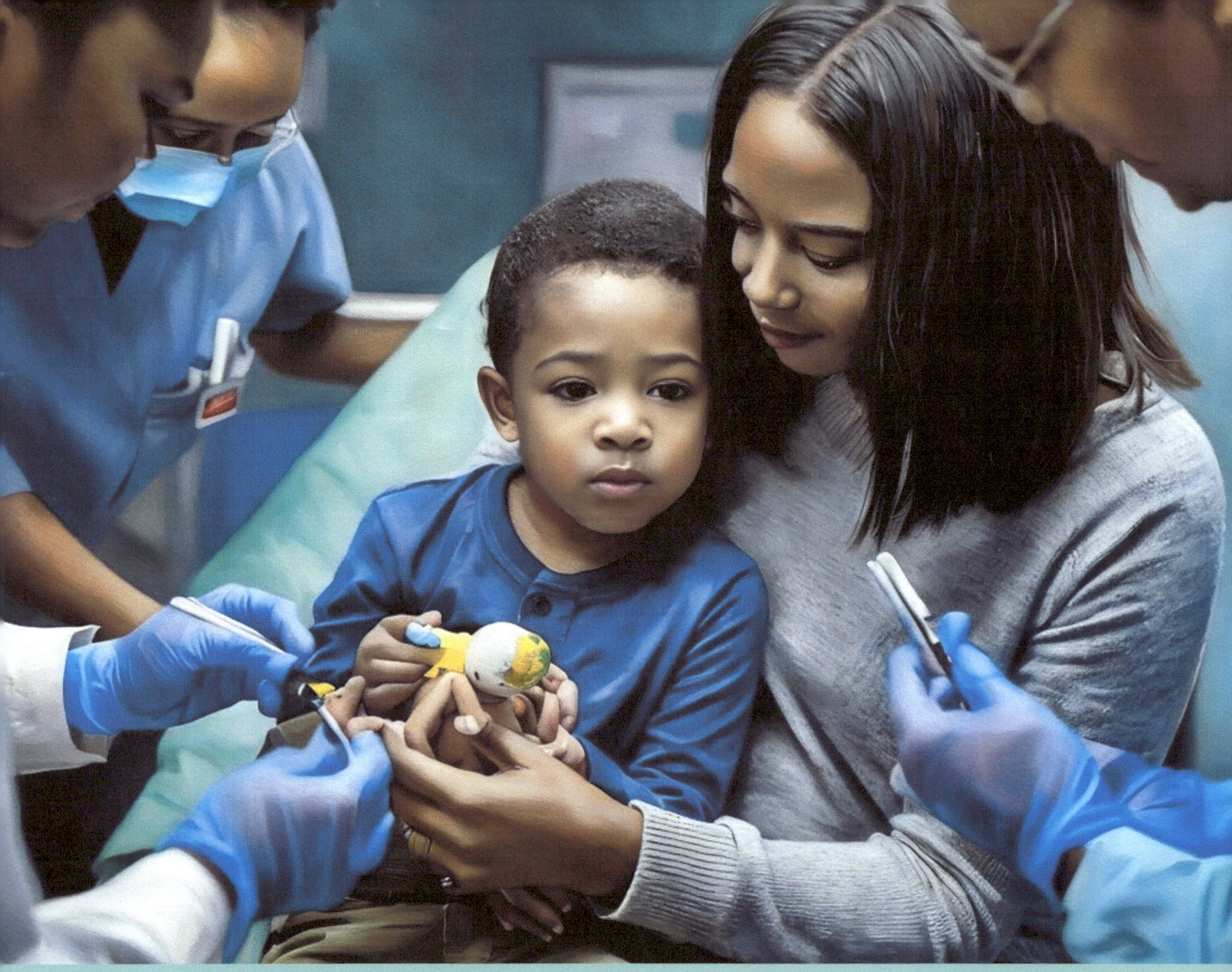

The doctor ran some tests and found out Karsen had Type 1 diabetes, and his kidneys were not working well. His mom held his hand and said, "You are so brave, Karsen."

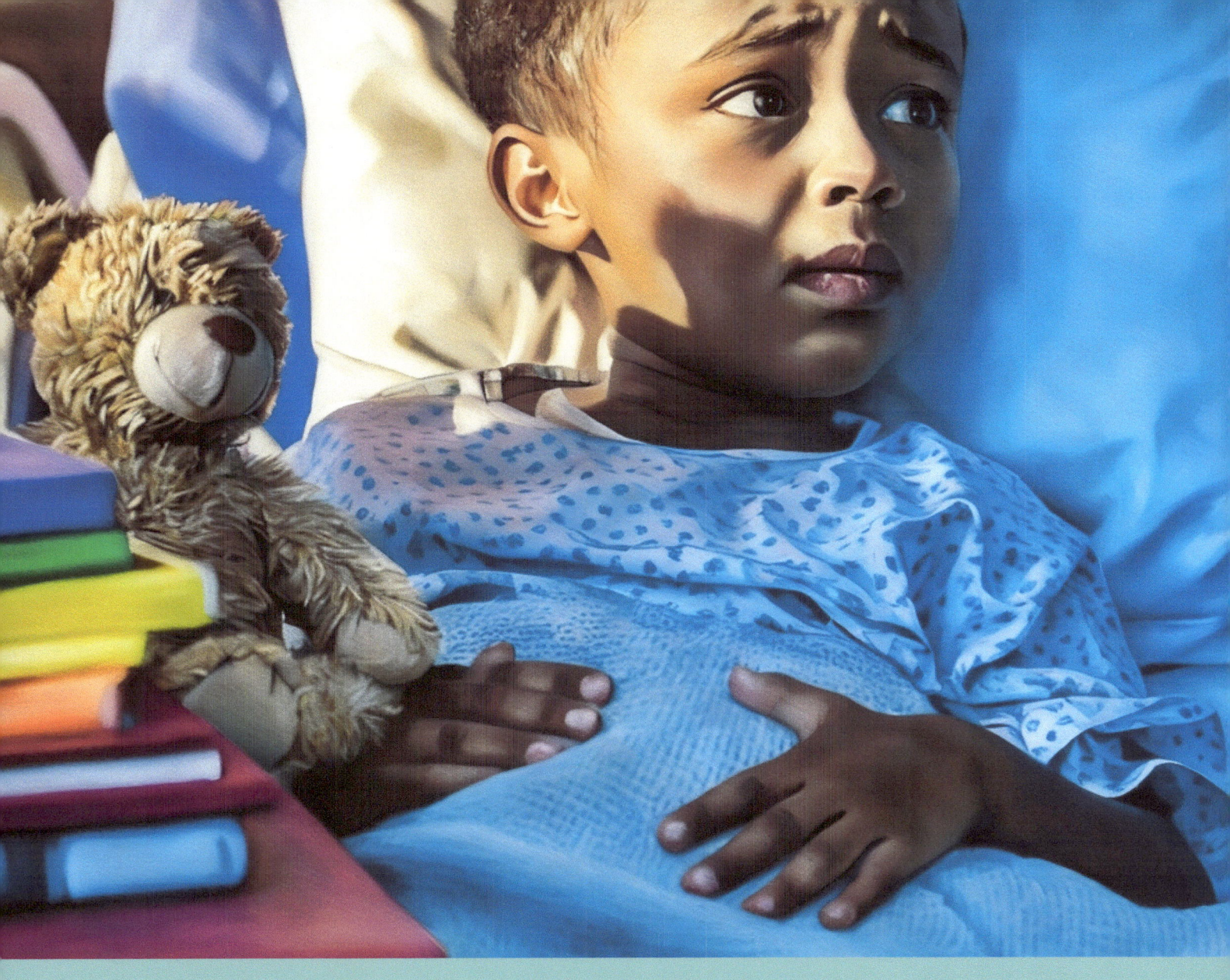

Karsen had to stay in the hospital for a few days.

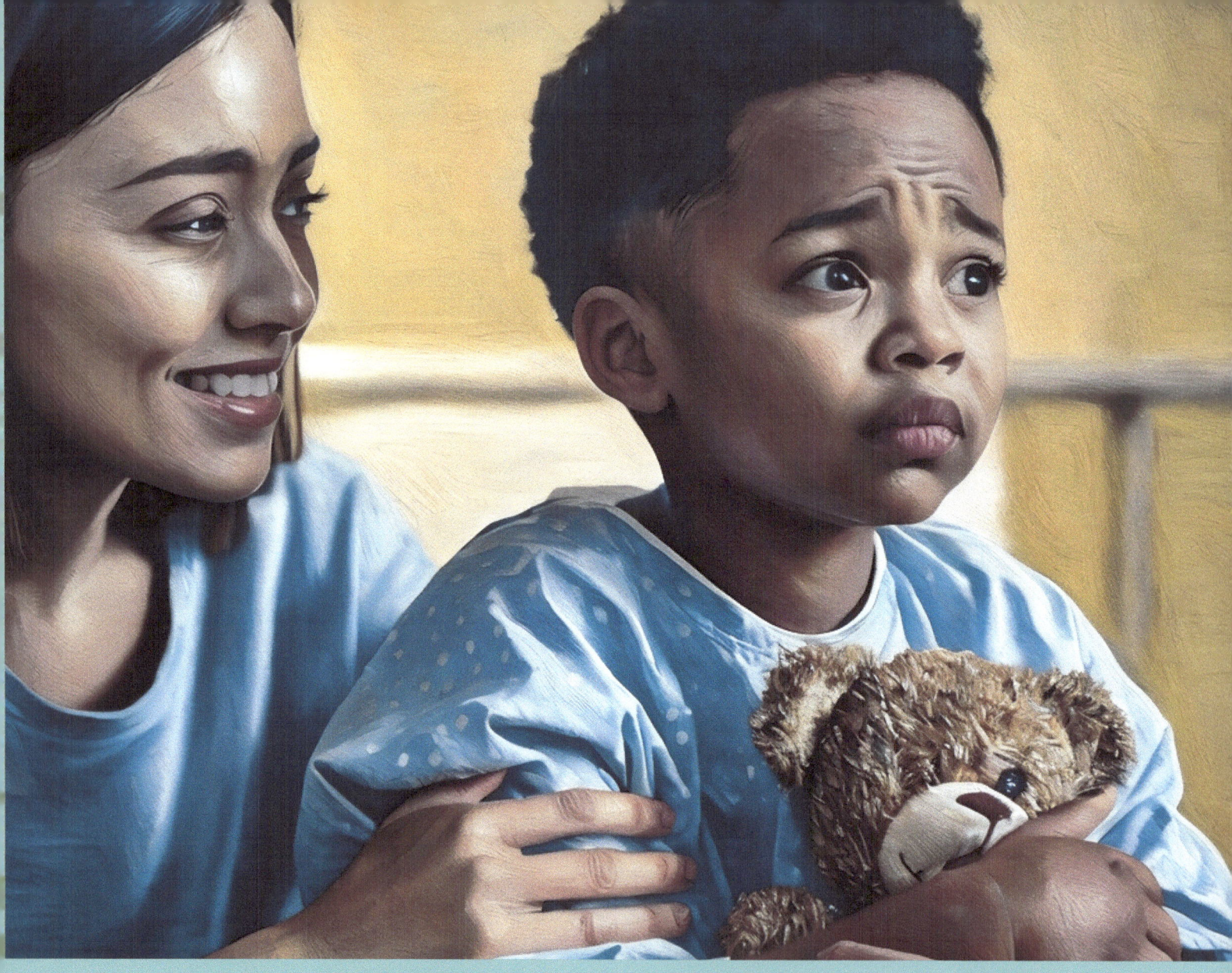

It was scary being in a new place, but his mom was always there, reminding her little warrior that he had a heart full of courage.

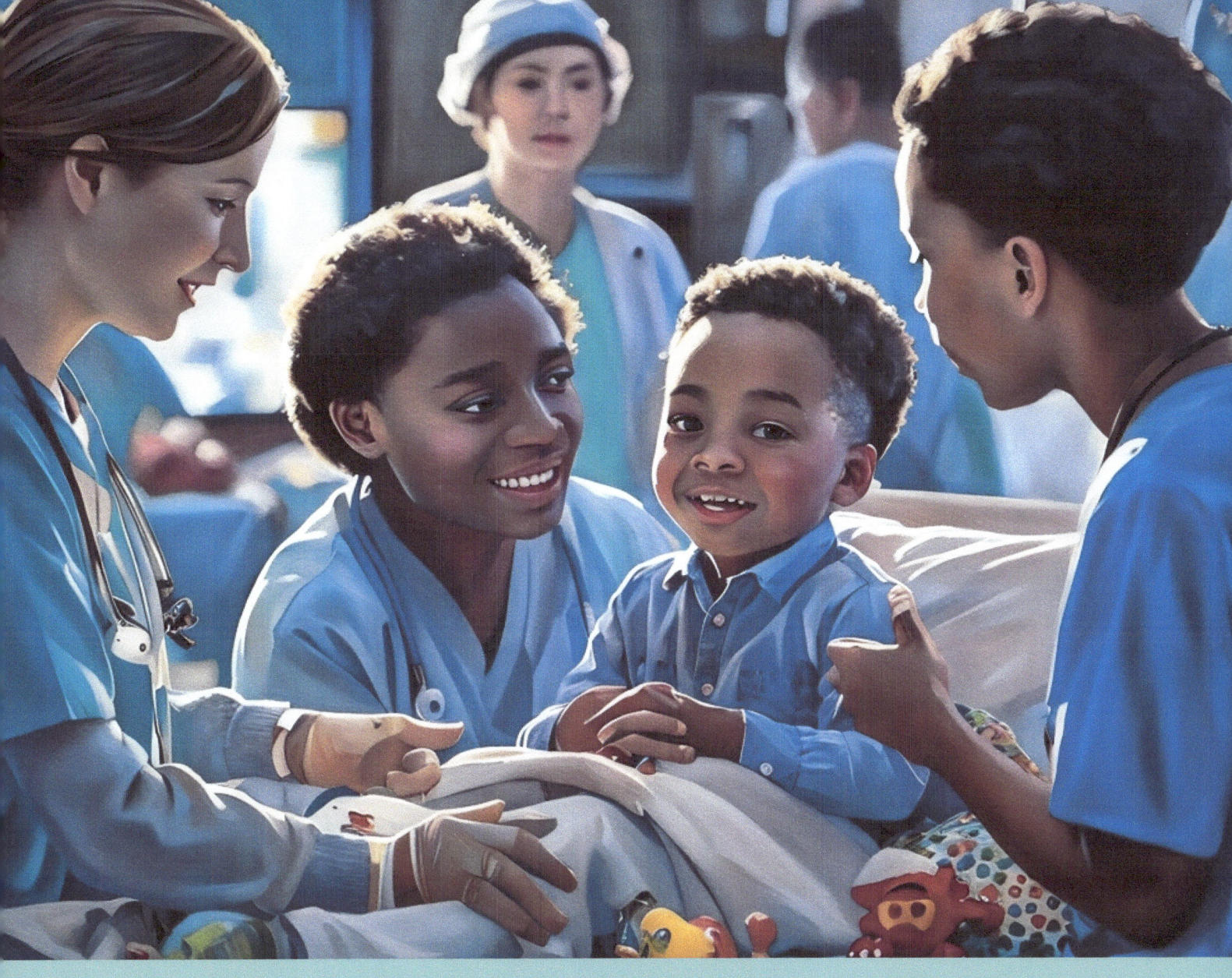

While they were in the hospital, a nice nurse named Sarah showed Karsen's mom how to check his blood sugar and use a new pen for his insulin.

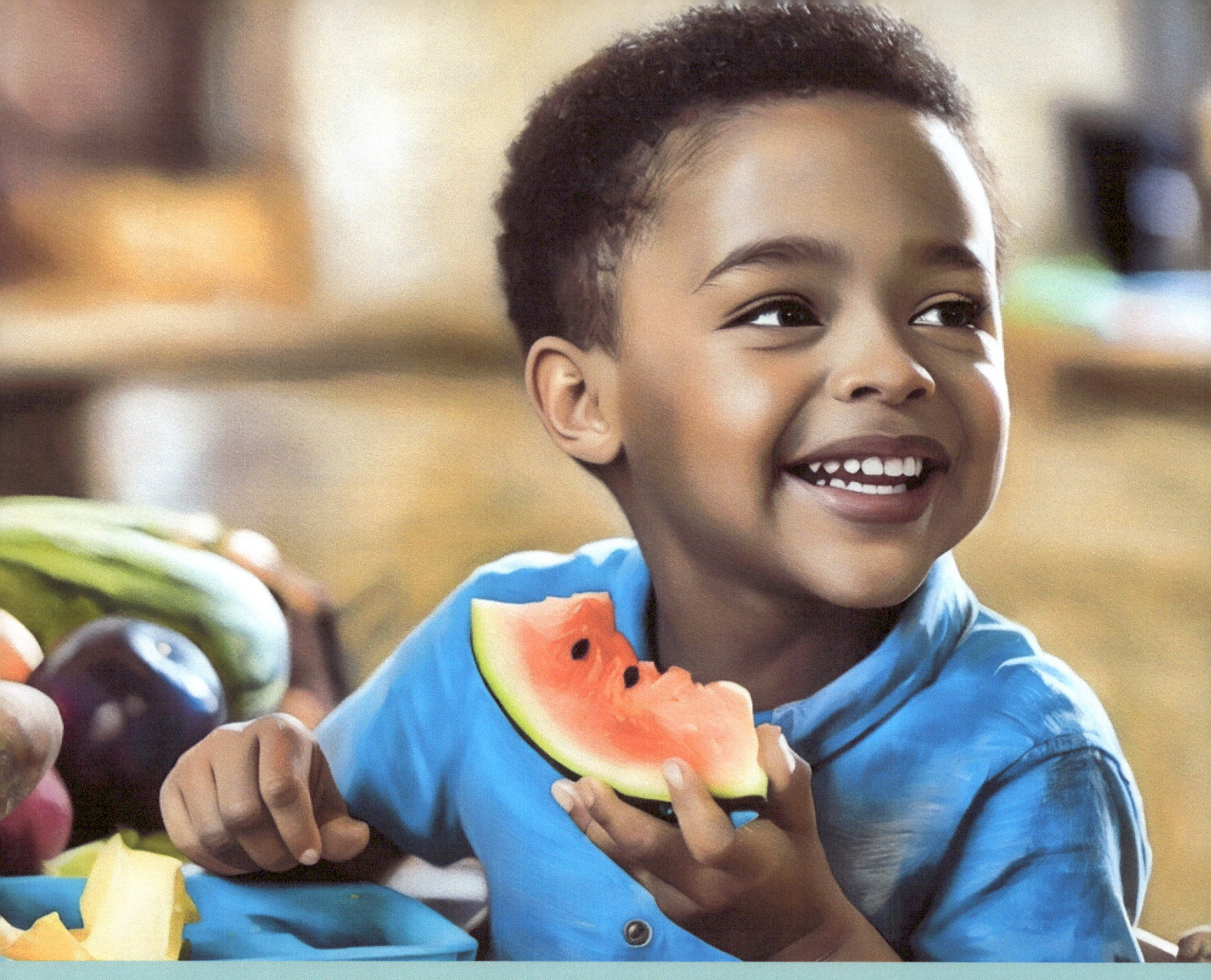

When they got home, Karsen had to start eating healthy foods and getting insulin every day.

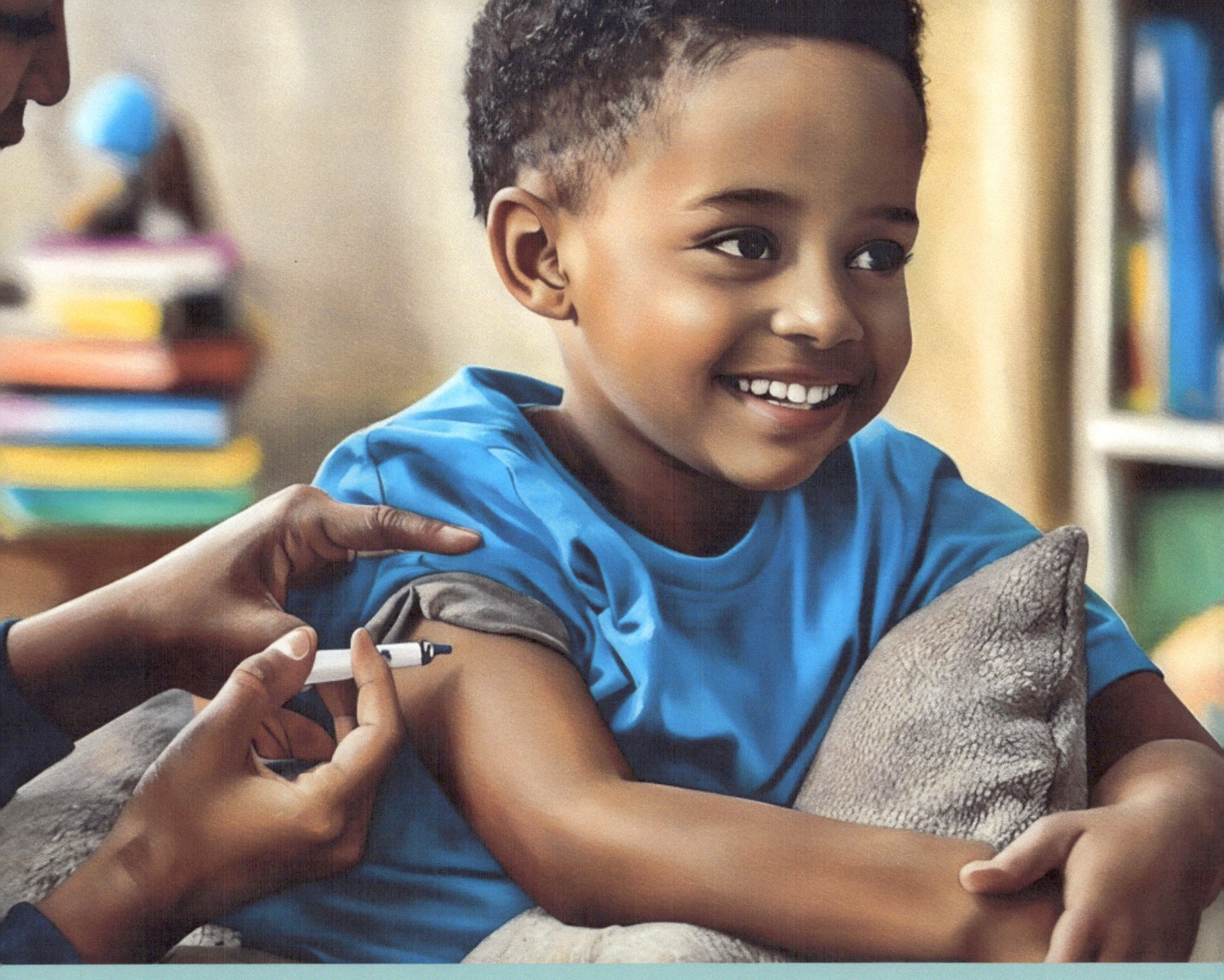

It was a big change for him, but his mom reminded him, "Every new step is a chance to show your amazing strength".

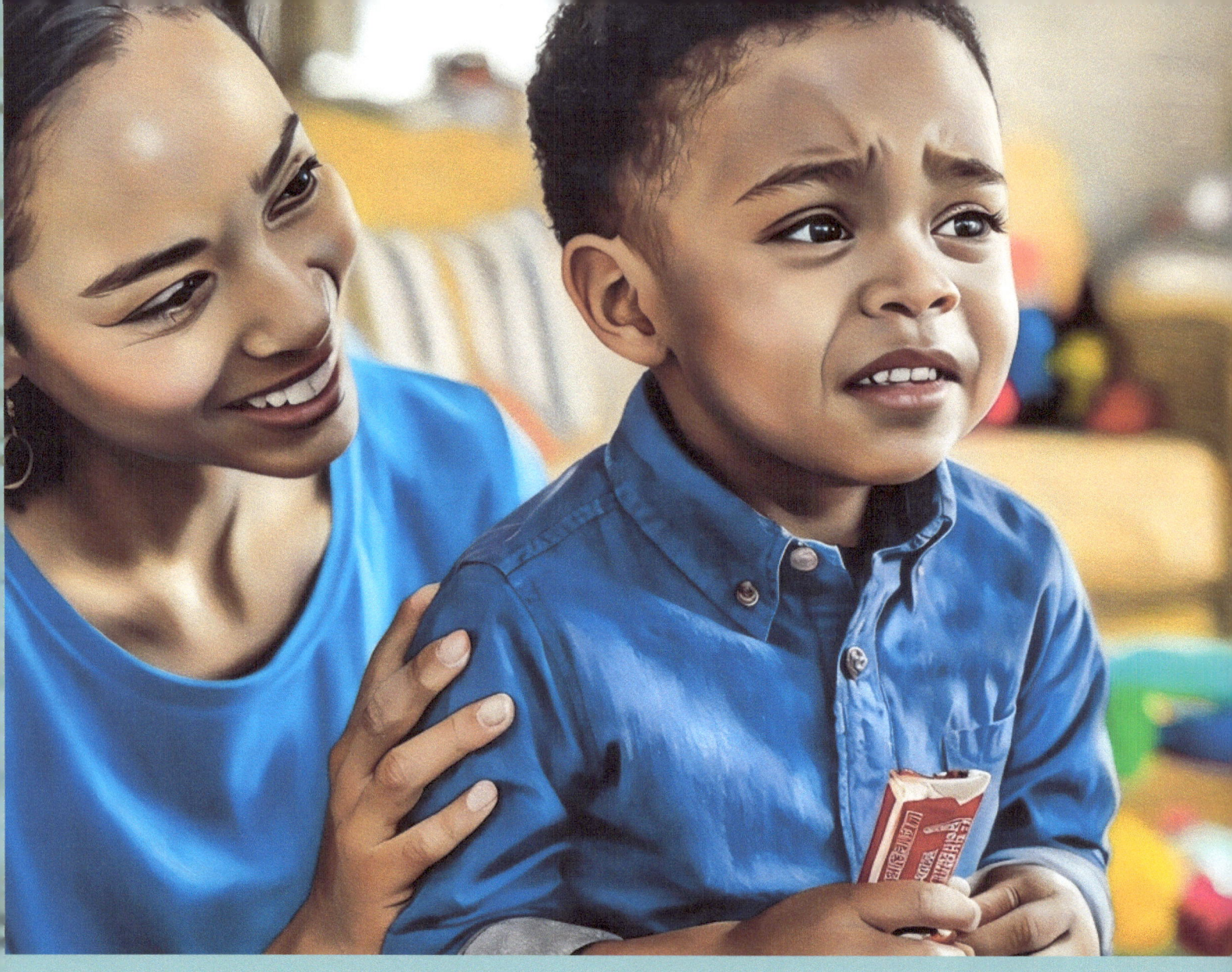

Sometimes Karsen felt upset because he couldn't eat his favorite snacks like he use to.

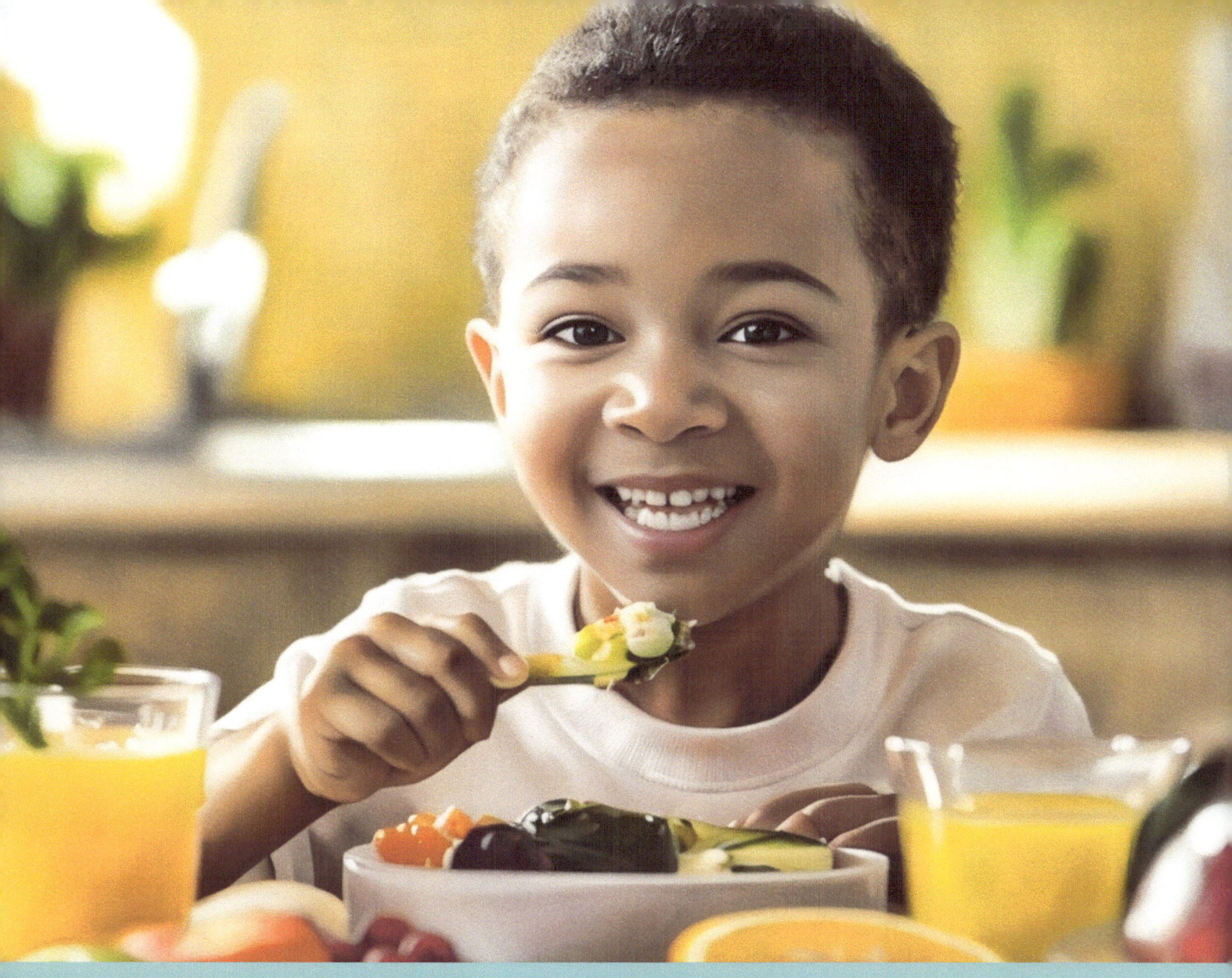

His mom helped him find yummy treats that were good for his body.

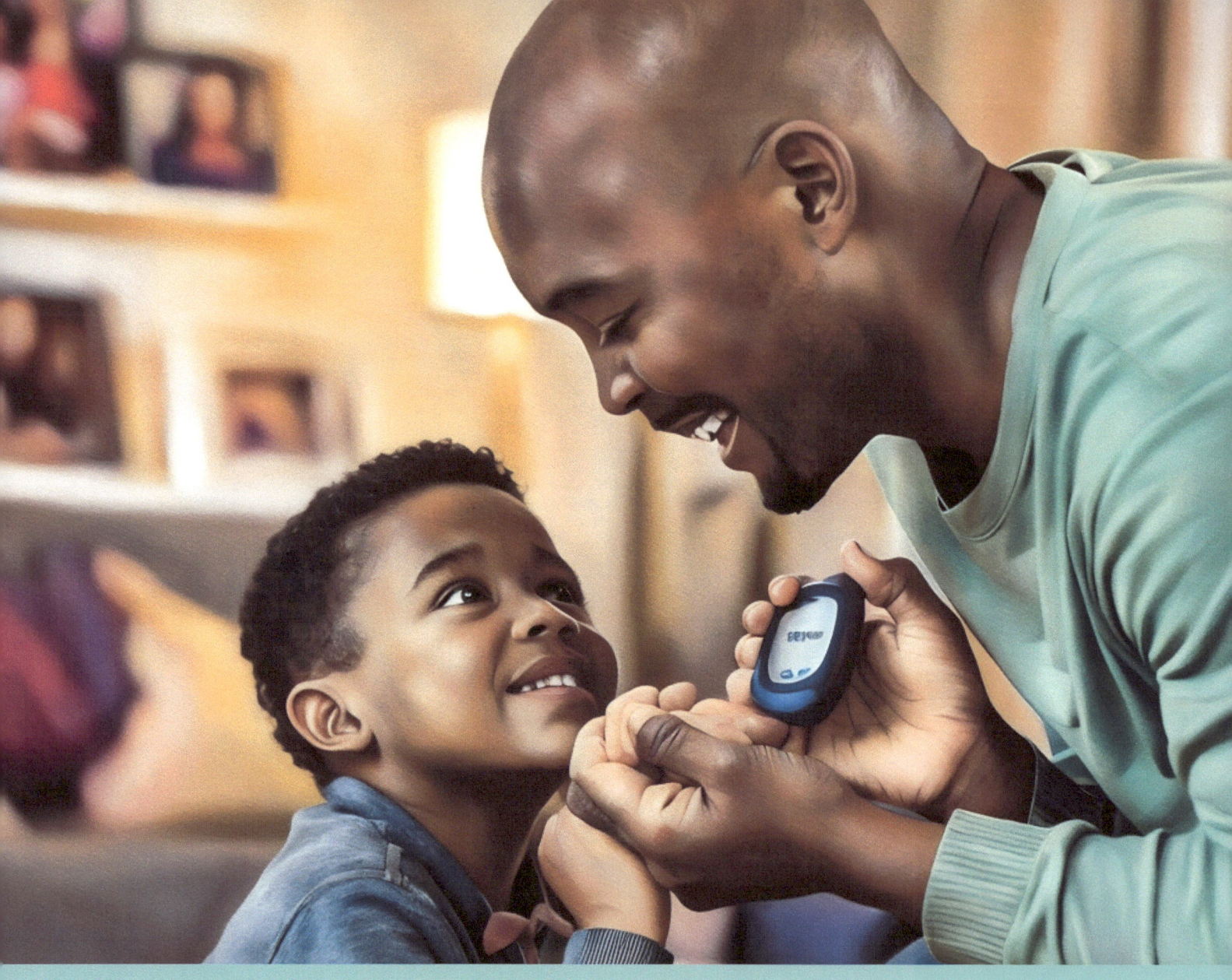

Karsen's big brother, Travis, made a special chart to keep track of Karsen's blood sugar levels. Travis said, "We are a team, Karsen, and together we can achieve anything."

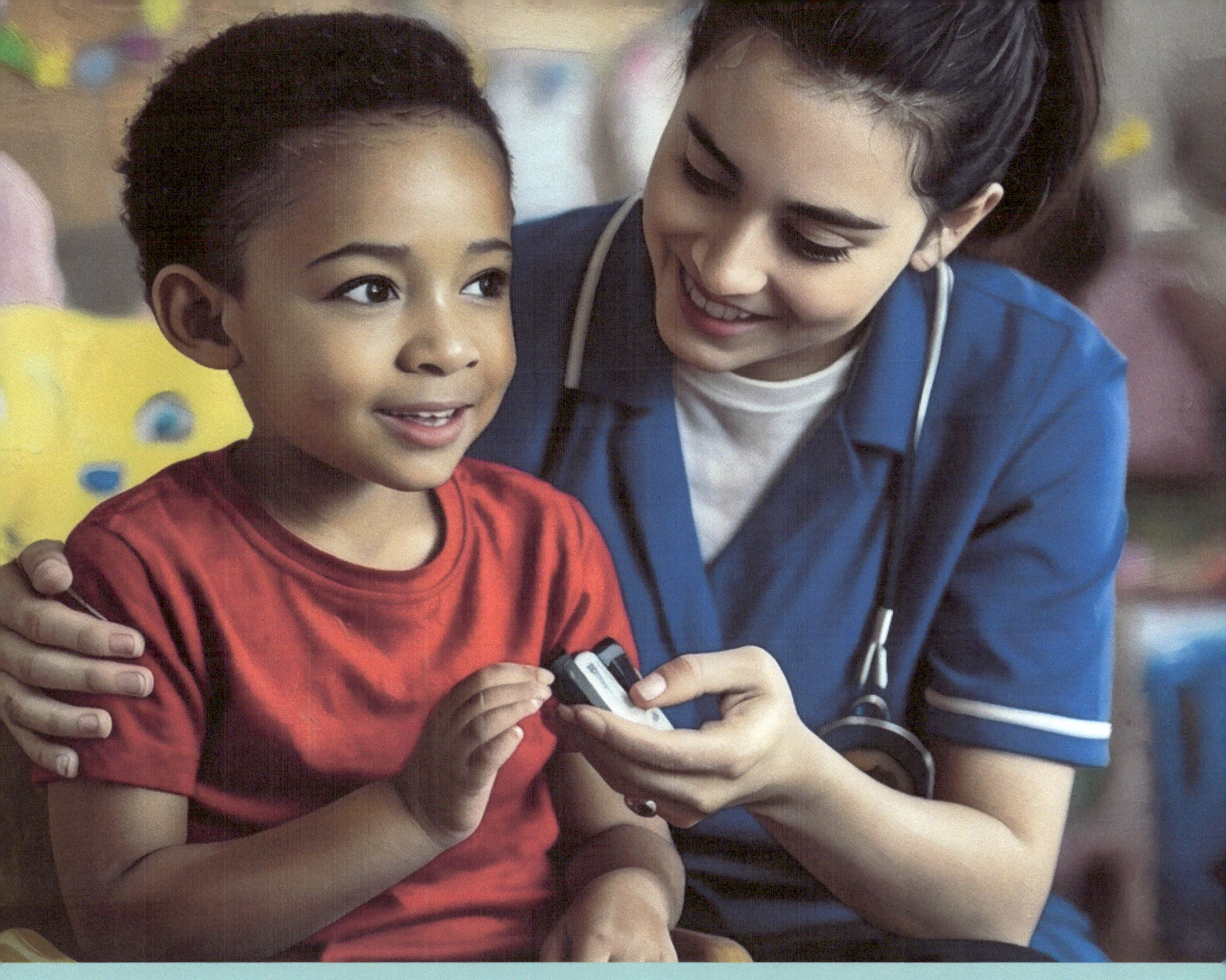

At home Karsen's nurse, Mrs. Lopez helped him by ensuring his glucose levels were below 200 and above 70.

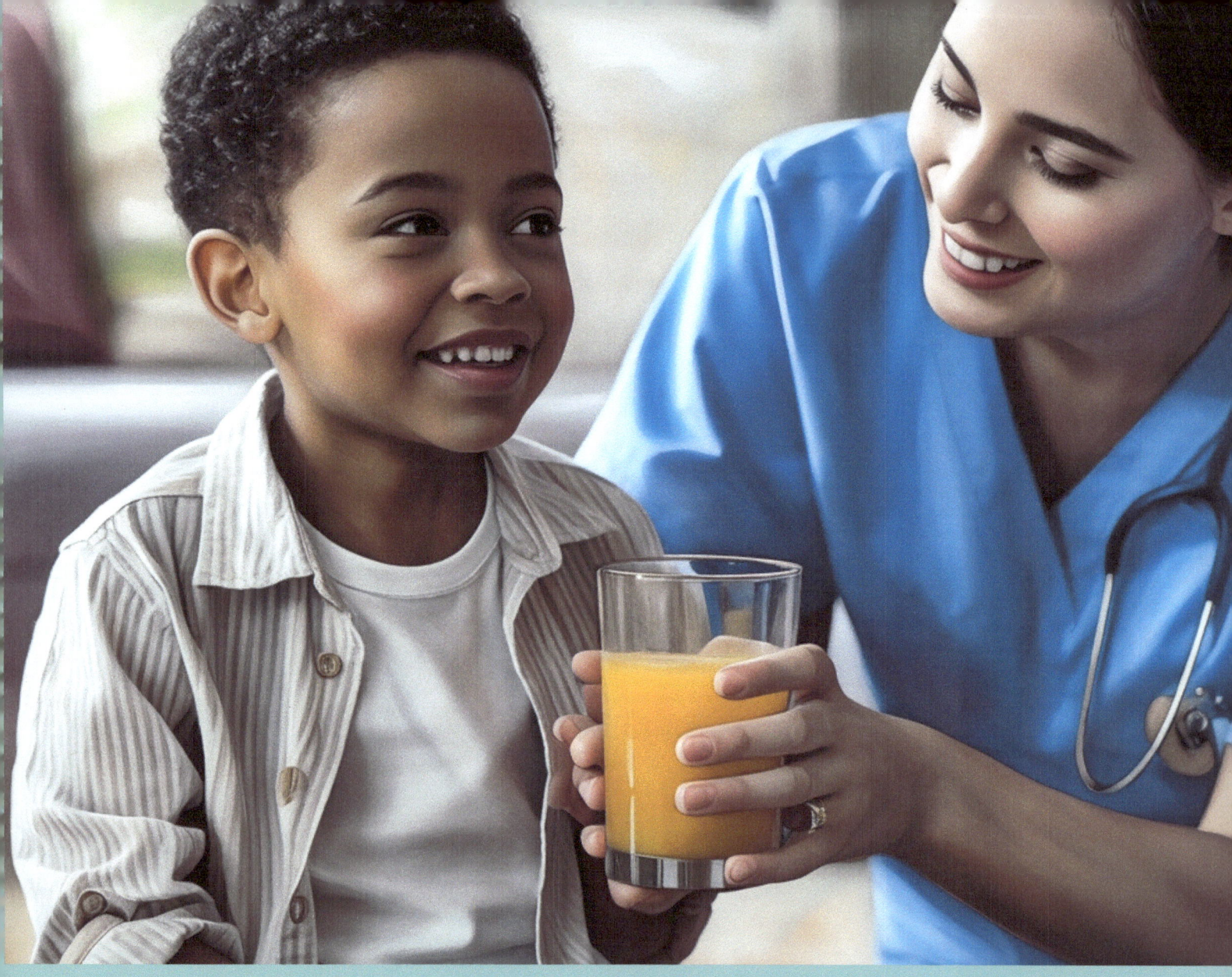

One day, Karsen blood sugar level fell below 70. Nurse Lopez knew just what to do. She checked his blood sugar and gave him a glass of orange juice to help him feel better.

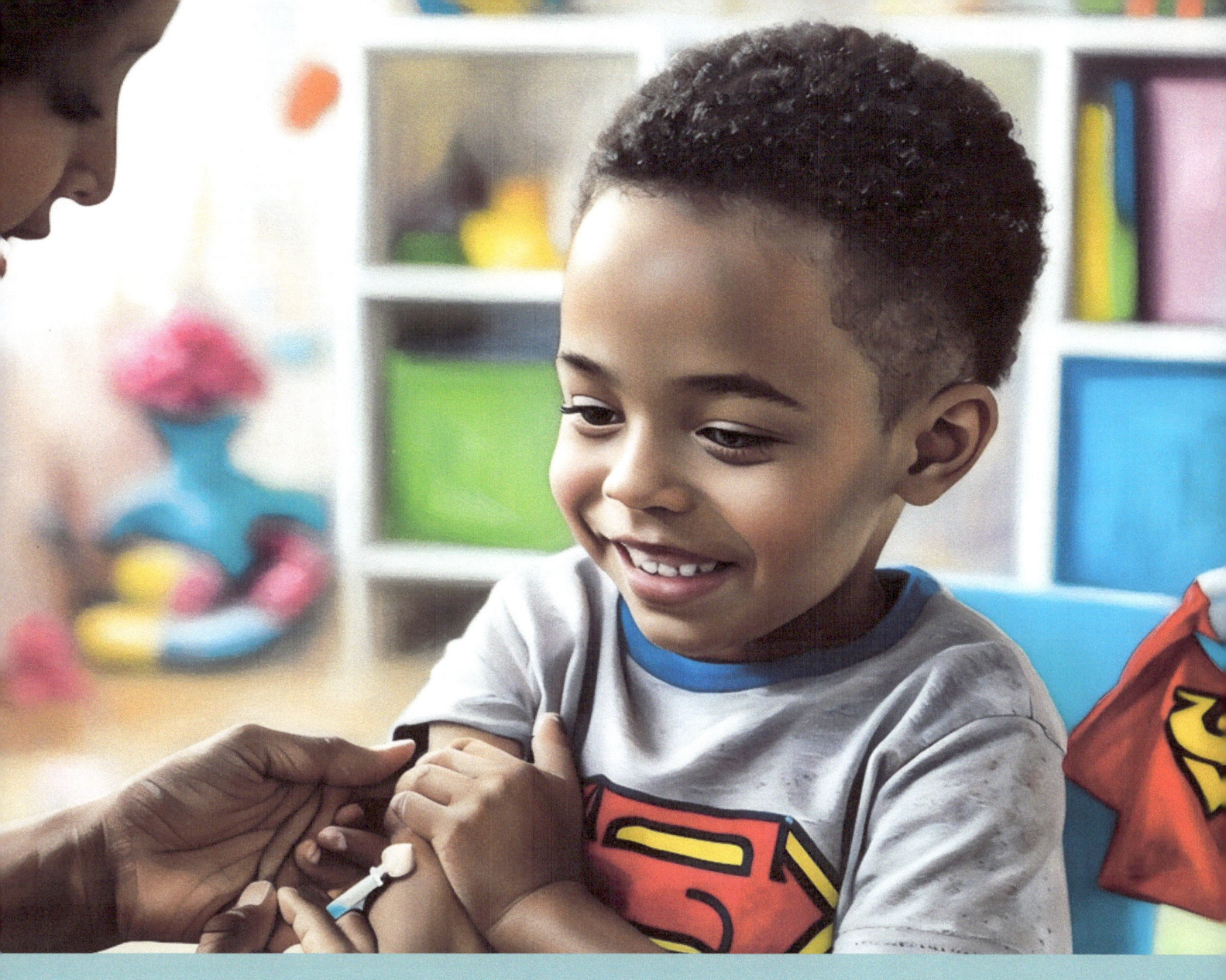

Karsen found it hard to get insulin injections every day.

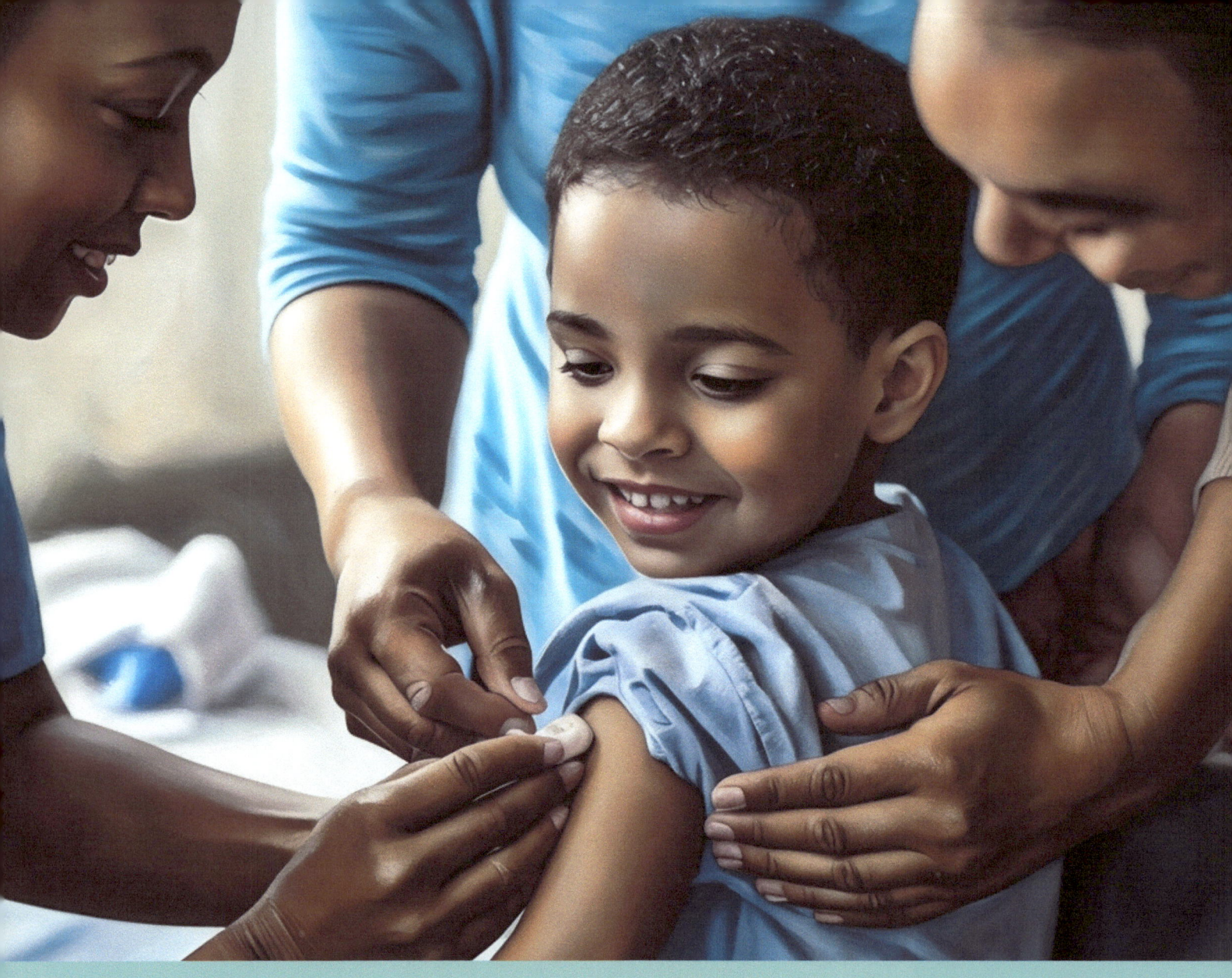

He got a cool new device called an Omnipod insulin pump. His mom said, "This pump is like your superpower, helping you stay healthy and strong."

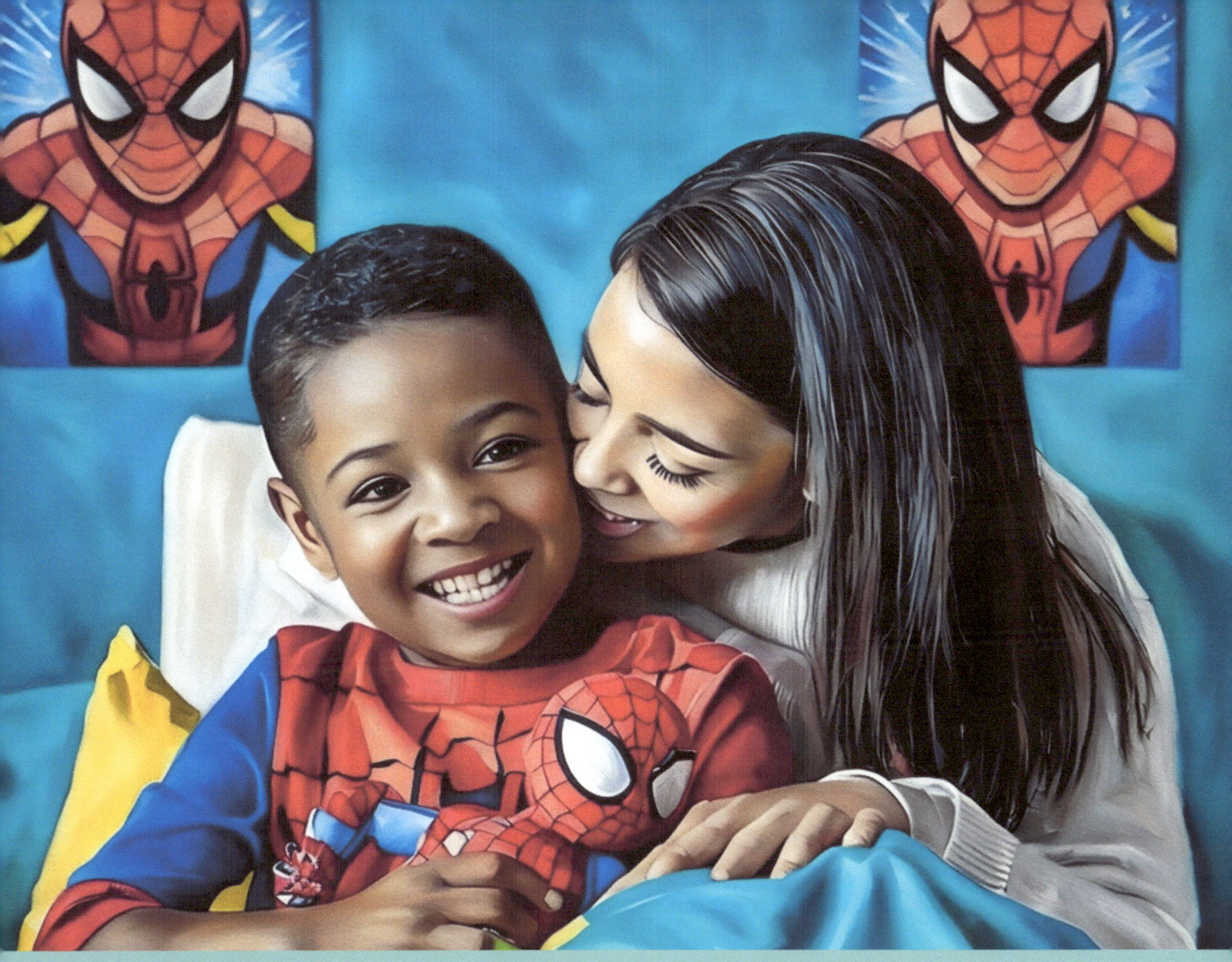

One night, Karsen's mom tucked him into bed and whispered, "I'm so proud of you, my brave boy." Karsen smiled, feeling warm and loved. He knew he was a true hero in his own story.

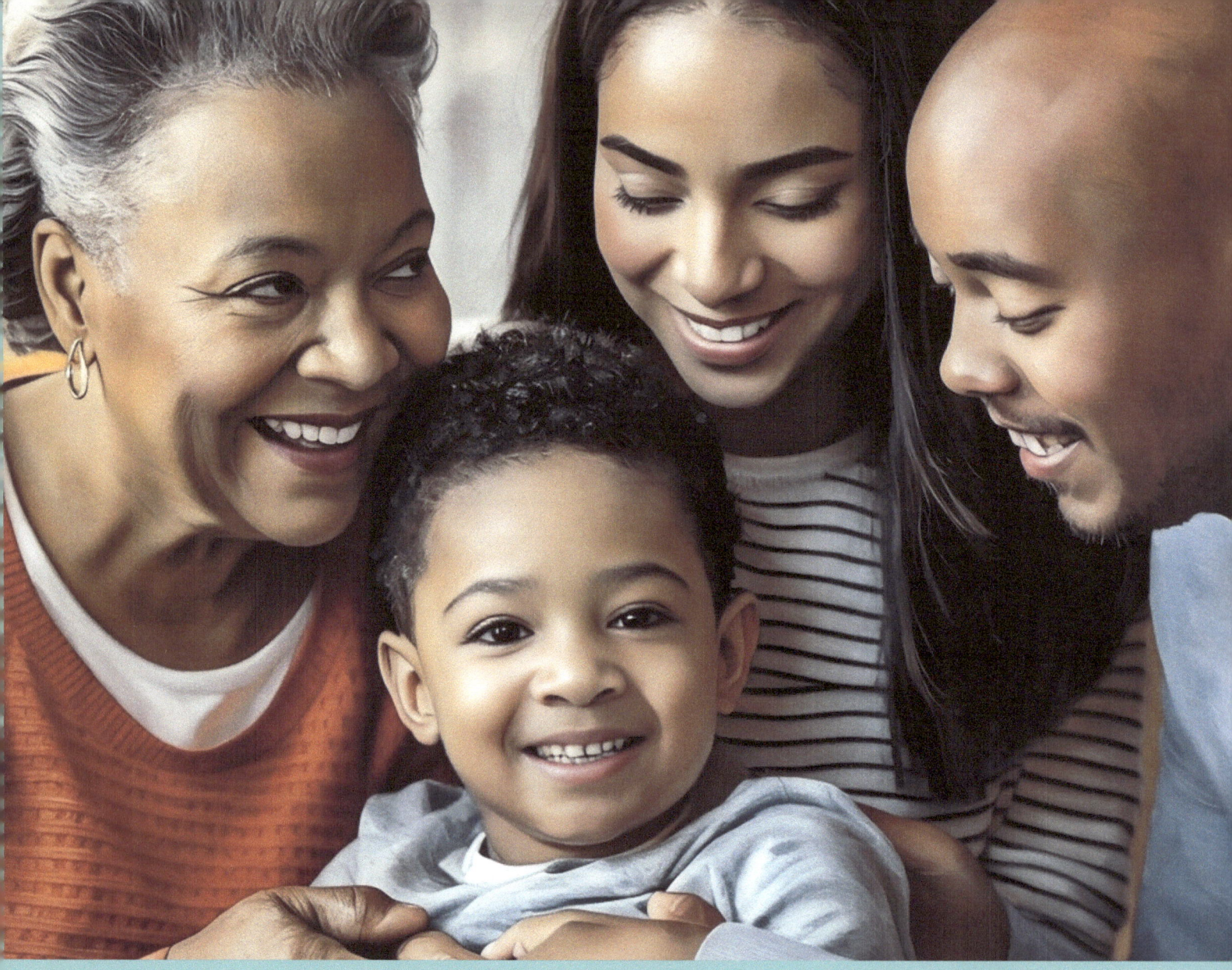

As the seasons changed, Karsen's family learned more about how to take care of him and his diabetes. They grew stronger together, finding joy in every little victory.

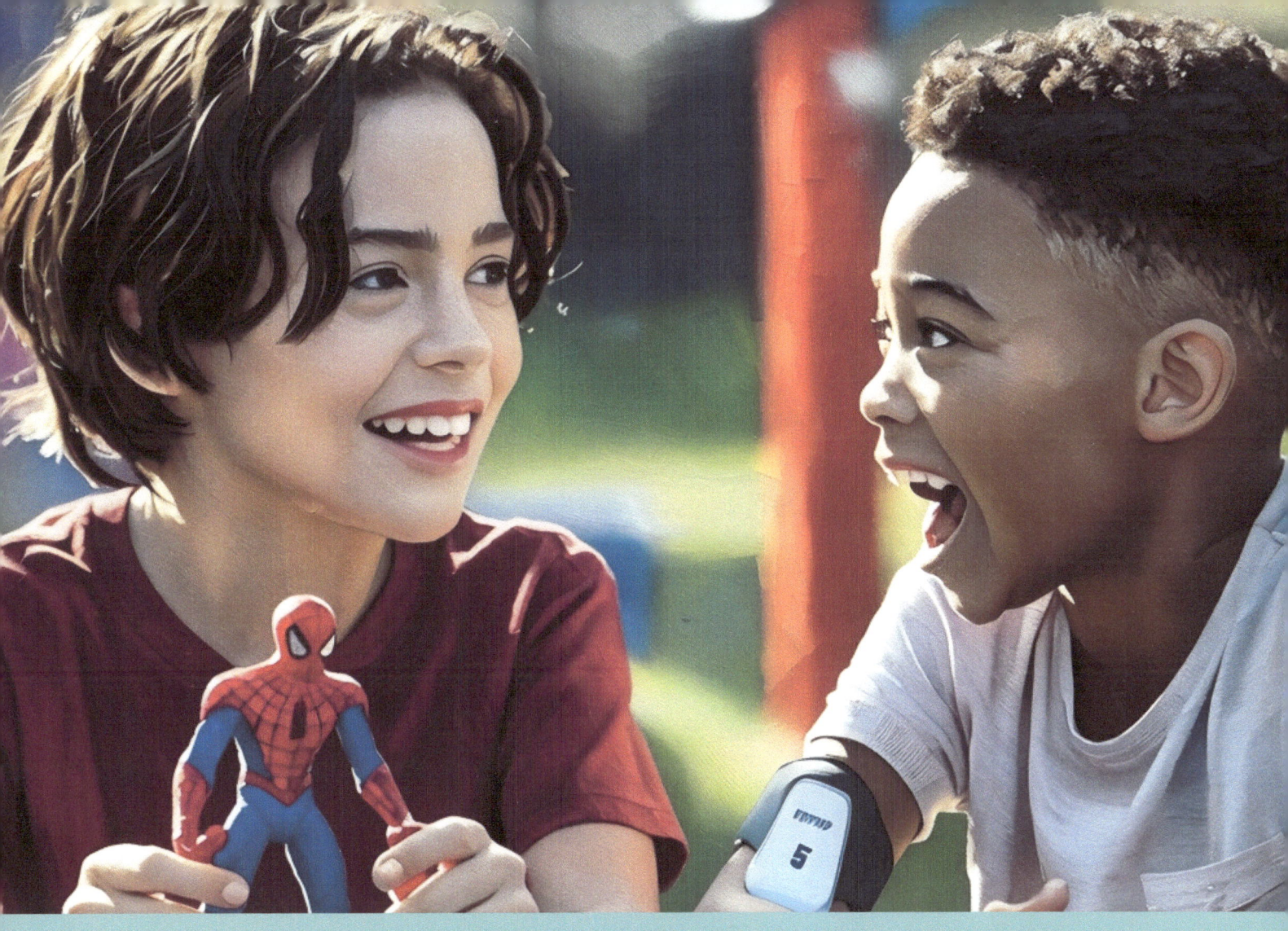

One sunny day at the park, Karsen met another boy who also had diabetes. They talked about their favorite superheroes. Karsen realized he wasn't alone and there were other kids just like him. He said to his new friend, "We are superheroes in our own special way."

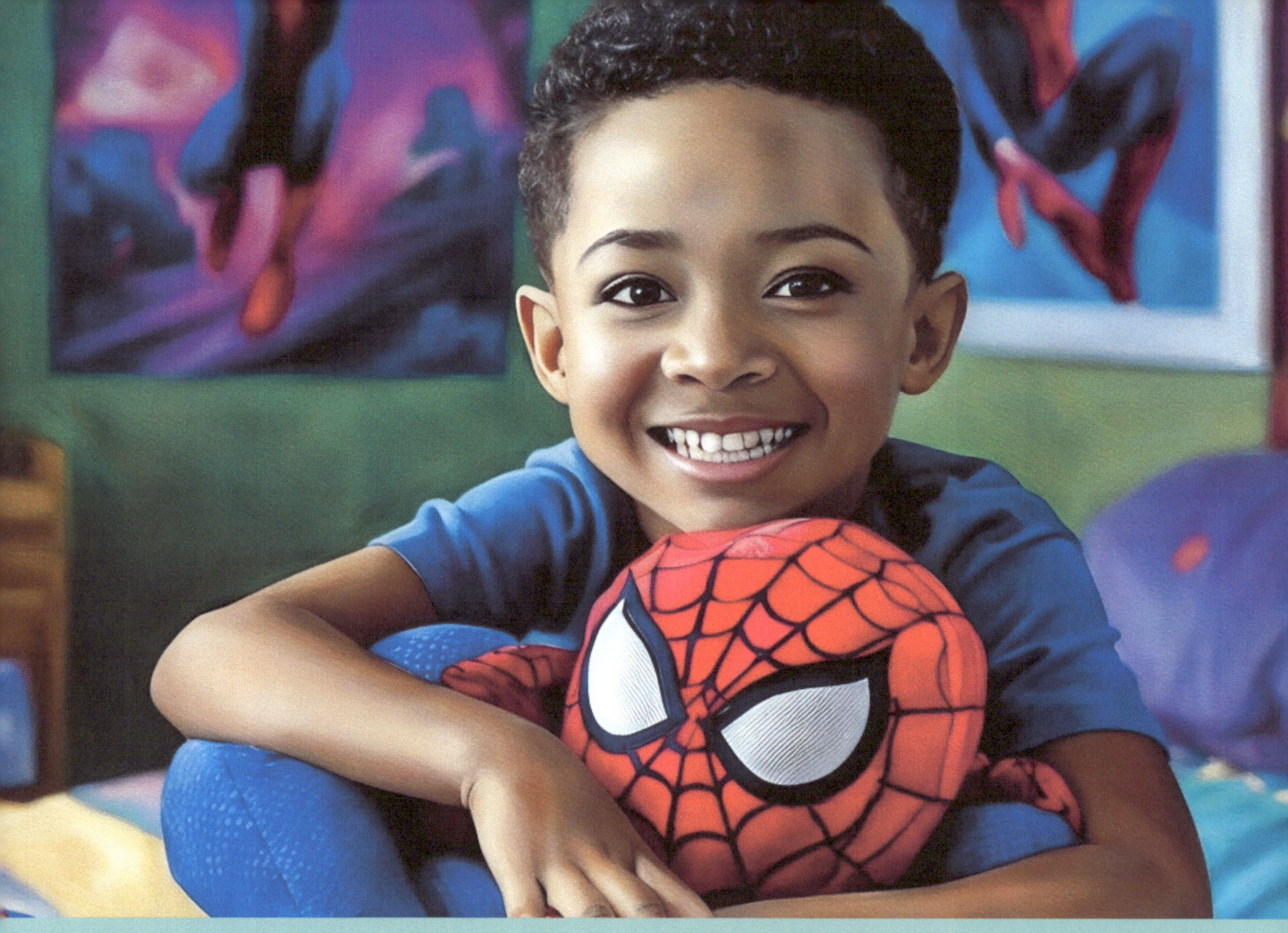

Karsen's journey was filled with challenges, but he faced each one with courage and strength. He learned that being a hero means never giving up and always believing in yourself. And every day, Karsen's story inspired others to be strong and brave, too.